Medical School, Your Plan B

Solid well paying jobs that are kept secret.

By Peter A. J.

Preface

Can anyone become a physician? Can anyone become a PGA golfer? I think so. But you better get ready for some real hard work. The thought of being a golfer on TV is much different than what it takes to be there. Statistics say that only 5% of golfers can break 80. Now what are the percentages to be a scratch golfer? That's a tall order that requires countless hours of study, practice, mental abilities with body aches and pains. Without a true love of golf, you can hang up your hat to the ranks of golf hacker. The exceptional fiery love of the sport will carry you through any ache and pain. So how do the PGA professionals do it? I've heard of just a few exceptional gifted players who attained such level simply by just reading a book and lots of hard work. However, the average Joe who does this without hard work, will barely break 100. To golf on TV, you need long hours of work, a personal coach who trains you step by step, and a true love for the sport.

Becoming a physician is quite similar; how much love do you really have for it? How much hard work are you willing to do and put up with?

It's a sad thought, but just my opinion: Computer video gaming is the modern opium. What a waste. I've seen kids waste learning opportunities from grammar school all the way through college. It has become highly addictive to the last few generations, destroying the fabric of what it means to work. Kids want to be "hooked up" into a good job, instead of busting their butt with good hard work.

Again, this is just my opinion.

The solutions I offer in this book will simply open doors for you. How much you bust your butt is up to you. Finally, I send truck-loads of gratitude to all those I have learned from, especially via osmosis. I may not be very intelligent, but I do listen and work hard.

Introduction

You can quickly open up page 37 and see all the secret jobs and their salaries.

Or you can slow down and not repeat past mistakes.

Contents of the Appendix

Let's Get Started

Ok, through no fault of your own, you are no longer a Resident, in medical school, or achieved a high MCAT.

Really………. no fault of your own?

Ok, I'm not going to lecture you on what a knuckle-head you are, or where you went wrong – In time you'll look back and have the real answer, not just the quick and dirty excuse of an answer you now give free rent inside your brain. Although, there are some of you who now find being a physician is just to darn tough to achieve. It's not your fault, remember that, ……… it's not your fault.

I think there is a genetic source that catapults some into being a physician, have you ever noticed that families of physicians usually have children who are physicians? It's like the nobility, you have to be born with blue blood. So, fate in it's wonderful mercy, has shown you that this family is not a good match for you. I'm always amazed when I read in the student medical forums, "I washed out I need a good Plan B" Then they grasp at anything and everything in desperate hope of salvaging what in the first place was not a successful match.

This book will examine why you chose to become a physician, and give you solid concrete alternative solutions.

- Remember Alfred and Batman?

"Master Bruce, why do we fall down?"

So we can learn how to pick ourselves back up!

Exactly! Now are you ready to pick yourself back up? Well I'm ready to show you, flip the page and let's get going!

Self Examination

Well, you signed up for medical school to examine others, when is the last time you examined yourself? In order to start this process we need a fair and honest evaluation. Step back, and look at yourself. What do you see?

Really?

What do you mean, step back and look at yourself?

I need a critical evaluation as to why you chose to become doctor. And don't give me those Cliff Note answers about working in a compassionate altruistic profession, where you can make a real difference.

Let's look at some reasons why

"I want to be a *Doctor*"

Money

Money

Money

Parents forced it on me

Status Symbol

To get married to another Doctor and have… more Money and live as a one percent-er.

To work with your hands and put bones back together.

To examine, diagnosis and find solutions.

To work with children because my Niece developed pneumonia at age two.

To work as a dermatologist because my Grandpa constantly scratches his legs.

To work in the ER, because my Mother was saved.

To work in the burn units, because my father fried himself at work.

To work with the C-Scope – well… for what ever reason.

Examine yourself and find the true reason why you wanted to become a " Doctor."

Only then will you be permitted to flip the page.

Find Your Candy

Did you know that students at Cal-Tech are told what classes they will take when they first enter? A student who entered as an aspiring astronomer, now finds out he's stellar in Chemistry. How did that happen? Well, in their infinite wisdom, Cal-Tech exposes the student to as many sciences as possible to find their perfect match.

Here's what they say:

Caltech will prepare you for the interdisciplinary nature of contemporary research in science and technology and position you for leadership roles in academia and industry. We include classes in the humanities and social sciences as an important component of the core curriculum to help you build effective written and verbal communications skills— essential no matter what field or profession you aim to enter. **(Caltech Undergraduate Admissions Page)** *https://www.admissions.caltech.edu/content/learning*

I remember the scientist across the street from my Uncle's house. He told me in the Philippines, being a physician was to be highly respected. So he entered The University of Santo Tomas. There he was exposed to Chemistry. The priests in their infinite wisdom directed him to a core curriculum in Chemistry because, "he read chem manuals like comic books."

This was his candy. He later went on to work for a major aerospace company in the states, helping to develop the ruby laser, bouncing it off the moon and so forth. He said he would go to work and dream. Get quiet and let the mind find solutions to his problems.

Tesla did that also, you know, the father of Alternating Current. Tesla would get quiet, pose a question, take a nap, then Bingo! The universal mind gave him a solution.

Let me tell you a little about myself. As a kid, I really had no idea about occupations. I just knew I liked drama, being on stage and playing in the levee. Then synchronicity took effect to put me in situations to achieve that. At age seven, some how my mother came across a boat load of costumes. We played Kings and Queens and make believe. In Middle school I took drama. I wanted to be the sheriff, but the director put me into the lead role as the singing cowboy in front of an entire auditorium. Drama and I continued in high-school and college. I remember acing college history essays because I would memorize them as four different scripts. I also became a stage magician having a ball. Truly, this was my candy.

Well, in high-school around the age of 16, I became aware of the facts of life and how as a matter of economics it would be a bit to uncomfortable making ends meet as a magician. So I shadowed my older cousin; he was studying to become an electrician. Thus, I took a fork in the road of life.

I became an electrician; but, soon found out that the Air-Conditioning Mechanic was a threat to my job, seeing that he did similar work. So I decided to enter High Voltage – that scared the daylights out of any A/C Mechanic. I knew this field would be stable. And it was. Later in my career, I found myself teaching through the Union in Texas at their Line Apprenticeship Program. It was right then and there when I knew I re-found my candy. It was very natural for me to get up on stage and present a lesson. Yes, I guess I do get a little dramatic, but it is a perfect match.

Perhaps you really enjoy the beach, the saltwater and sun. I remember one job I had – Container Crane Electrician Port of Houston. I was brand new on the job; they threw me to the wolves. The crane was out of order, and I had to get the boom lowered. Now, not to many people know this, but if the boom over speeds on the way down, the whole thing will topple over into the ocean. They informed me about this and left me there with another Green-horn. Well, we worked around the clock and eventually repaired it. In the morning we looked out onto the ocean and saw the sun rising from a smooth piece of glass salt water. No matter how much they threw at me, it didn't matter - it was a perfect environment.

Dr. Robert Ballard, who found the ship Titanic, was born in 1942. He truly has found his candy. Still in excellent shape, he said he desires to continue to search under water for the rest of his life."*The most important discoveries were the ones I didn't know were there,*" he says. "*I can only tell you that we've looked at so little, there has to be huge discoveries still waiting for us,*" (2015 Interview with CBS 60 Minutes) This guy refuses to retire, that's the best job in the world.

What I'm trying to say is to have a successful career, something that is truly rewarding, you have to find what really turns you on.

Read as many autobiographies as possible. These are great people who are trying to teach us so we can have a shortcut in life.

Review your life, were there things in synchronicity that you were really not aware of?

Perhaps these will give insight as to your new Plan B.

Move out of my way!

I want to be the boss. I am going to run this place. I will be in charge of a multi-million dollar corporation. I want to live high on the hill. I want a show case wife, have two kids, drive a 911 Carrera. I worked my ass off – damn it, I finally deserve it. After all he who dies with the most toys wins – Right?

Well, I guess so. But maybe not. I believe it's how you got there to that position in life that is more important. Did you rise to the top by reading, "The Art of War." Or did you keep persisting, never giving up, always with the thought – what can I do to help others?

Peter Cooper is an excellent role model. An entrepreneur, had tons of money and a very unique philosophy in life – to be in service. I found an online book (openlibrary.org) By Charles Edwards Lester that talks about the life and character of Peter Cooper. It's worth the read. He, like Tesla, had the unique ability to tap into the Universal Source of knowledge for service of others. The more he gave, the richer he became. Hmmmmmm, sounds pretty good, I'd like a job like that. It's all about intentions. Examine your intentions. I scrounged around and found some interesting work quotes.

"Failure is another steppingstone to greatness."

— Oprah Winfrey

"We often miss opportunity because it's dressed in overalls and looks like work" — Thomas A. Edison

"I'm a greater believer in luck, and I find the harder I work the more I have of it"

— Thomas Jefferson

"No one who does good work will ever come to a bad end, either here or in the world to come"

— The Bhagavad Gita

"If you trust in yourself. . .and believe in your dreams. . .and follow your star. . . you'll still get beaten by people who spent their time working hard and learning things and weren't so lazy."

— Terry Pratchett, *The Wee Free Men*

"Be steady and well-ordered in your life so that you can be fierce and original in your work."

— <u>Gustave Flaubert</u>

"The great secret of true success, of true happiness, is this: the man or woman who asks for no return, the perfectly unselfish person, is the most successful."

— <u>Swami Vivekananda</u>

" There are no secrets to success. It is the result of preparation, hard work, and learning from failure."

— <u>Colin Powell</u>

"Talent is cheaper than salt. What separates the talented individual from the successful one is a lot of hard work."

— <u>Stephan King</u>

"Choose a job you love, and you will never have to work a day in your life."

— Confucius

"Out of clutter, find simplicity."

— Albert Einstein

"The less you need, the happier you are."

— **Peter A.J.**

By the Hour

I spent some time at Salary.com and other sites to find out exactly how much does a physician in my neighborhood makes. So at the time of this writing (2015) here is what I found.

Physician Family practice: $ 189,000
Surgeon : $ 400,000

These are the annual salaries. Yes, set salaries, no overtime pay, does not include items such as:

Required meetings, insurance, cost of litigation, preparing medical records, clinical reports and correspondences, time spent after hours to maintain certification.

I found this online Washington Post:
http://www.washingtonpost.com/news/to-your-health/wp/2014/05/22/how-many-patients-should-your-doctor-see-each-day/

In an email, Lou Goodman, president of the foundation, wrote that "*physicians are working fewer hours, seeing fewer patients and limiting access to their practices in light of the significant changes to the medical practice environment. The research estimates that if these patterns continue, 44,250 full-time-*

equivalent physicians will be lost from the work force in the next four years."

He predicted that within the next three years, *"more than 50 percent of physicians will cut back on patients seen, work part-time, switch to concierge medicine, retire or take other steps likely to reduce patient access."*

With millions of people newly insured under the Affordable Care Act, patients may face even more challenges finding access to doctors. About 75 percent of the doctors in the survey described themselves as *"overextended and overworked"* or *"at full capacity,"* about the same who said that in 2008. But 58 percent said they spend zero to 10 hours on paperwork each week, and 26.1 percent said they spend between 11 and 20 hours on those duties each week.

After all the number crunching A family practice physician makes about $60 / hour.

How bout all those bills you have to repay? Student loans, auto, rent, lawyers, now how much do you have left over to save?

Ah, you say. That's why you have to specialize – to make the big bucks.

This is true.

But that's for people who have exceptional skills and genetics that allowed them to progress to that height.

Now think about this :

The riskier a job is, the greater the pay.

Can you live with leaving sponges inside the belly or gassing someone to death?

Well, there are safety checks and measures physicians take to ensure that the odds of doing so is greatly reduced. However, complacency will always make you famous, in a bad way.

That brings me to your Plan B.

In the Industry most wages are paid by the hour. Anything over your 40 hrs / week is paid in overtime: time and a half and double-time. Depending on the industry, some jobs have a considerable amount of overtime. During emergencies it's not unheard of to double your salary. Can you guess it? Yup – the High Voltage Industry.

Typically, jobs like these set you up for an excellent retirement: 401K, Deferred Comp, an actual retirement pension, vacation time, sick pay, health / medical benefits,   AND TUITION REIMBURSEMENT.

At the moment the High Voltage Industry is in a tight jam – we don't have enough workers to do the jobs nation wide. Why is that? They call it, "The Silver Tsunami."

All those baby boomers who occupied these skilled positions have/or are retiring. Our apprenticeship program typically hires 15 students per year. We now are hiring two classes of 15 per year due to the shortage.

A high-school grad, with high voltage electrical experience can qualify and pull down $89,000 per year, while attending the apprenticeship program.

WHAT? Getting paid to go to school? - Exactly. That's what an apprenticeship program is all about. After graduation, the apprentice becomes a Journeyman, making over $100k per year. Depending on what and where the job is at, a Journeyman can double that with overtime. However, there are draw-backs, you are never home working all those hours. So for a family guy, all those hours are not so cool. Electricians of all trades are trained to perform CPR and use the AED. This is not just someone buckling over in the office. This is full emergency, pull-top rescues to save your tool buddy who just made contact.

Perhaps you are a lady who did not make the grade, or a man who just does not like to get so dirty. Look up **Electric Substation Operator**. This is a thinking job where you must switch in and out electrical equipment as big as a garage. Perform the wrong switching, you can drop an oil refinery or other critical equipment. That being said, they constantly receive training, to drill in those safety checks and procedures to keep accidents to a minimum. Is there an acceptable level – none. However, once you do become an operator, you can then promote to being a **System Operator** controlling the whole city. Glass ceiling?– not for women. The System Operator is a pressure cooker of a job, that demands concentration more powerful than a laser. The hours are long and the overtime is tremendous. Now what do you think?

A lot of hard work, ...yup.

Is the work dangerous, ...yup.

Dirty, ...yup

Working with tools, ...yup.

Will you sweat and sometimes get stinky, ...yup.

Could you die?... If you become complacent.

If you want to see some video's of electrical workers and blow ups – search YouTube for "Arc-flash"

There is risk in flipping hamburgers, there's risk in catching the plague as a research PhD. I would rather risk electrical burns and high pay over getting burned flipping hamburgers for low pay.

Remember I said the more riskier a job is the more it pays? Here are a few West Coast examples of base wages **without overtime included.**

Electrical Substation Operator: $102K, equipment blowing up near you, dropping an oil refinery.

Electrical Substation Mechanic: $102K, electrical contact

Lineman: $120K, cutting out and falling off a pole, electrocution

System Operator: $145K, dropping the entire city, all dark. Base rate = 75% of Family Practice

Electrical Engineer: $150K, miscalculations can cost millions. Base rate = 79% of Family Practice

Executive Electrical Manager: $250 to 300k, some companies well past $1 Million

Here is a story:

Instructor Jack P. had a student with an exceptional IQ.

"What a pain in the butt he was, but somehow he listened to me and targeted System Operator. He entered as a Substation Electrician Trainee, then spent three years after graduation, as a Journeyman. He took the System Operator exam, and made it past probation."

That was unheard of! The S.O. job is tough as nails for operators. So, anything is possible if you really set your mind to it and work hard.

Exam? Did I say exam?

The Exam

Yes.

To get any kind of Civil Service or industry position you have to take an exam, then do a six month probation. There *are* study guide books available on just about every Civil Service job out there at the library or bookstore. Each job has a job posting that details the pay, job duties, requirements, and WHAT WILL BE ON THE EXAM. Do you know how many people don't read that part – a lot. Some exams are 100% interview. How high you score on your exam is paramount to your success, especially if there are a limited amount of positions. Don't wait for the exam bulletin to be published before you start to study. This will only give you two weeks to study. Make a visit to Human Resources or get online and grab an old bulletin. Now you have time for a complete preparation.

When the exam is published, you'll have to fill out an application. Fill in every single space, no fudging with white lies. That move can later be used to fire you. Sometimes H.R. will notify you that they lost your application. This will be easy because you already made a copy of the app, or print screened and saved it to file. Now, this will ensure you have a matching application.

Do all your studying way before the exam – months. Keep a strong physical fitness program or your brain will turn to mush. The 24 hour period before the exam – just relax no studying.

You will receive an exam time and exam location. Google map it and find out with street view exactly where the parking lot is. Get there way early so you can have choice parking, time to eat some veggies for mental alertness, and time to find a restroom for a very nervous poop.

Once taking the exam, read each question carefully, along with all answers. It's easy to grab a correct answer staring at you, however there may be more than one correct answer. A common trick is for the test maker to have wrong answers based upon incorrect methods. For example: You have worked out the Power calculation for a three phase circuit, see your answer and grab it fast. However, it is flat wrong, you forgot to multiply your answer by 1.73 to account for three phase.

Ensure answer # 20 goes to question #20. It's easy to fail an exam if you are one number off. After you complete the exam, and if you still have extra time, go walk to the restroom and wash your face with cold water. Do some toe touches and knee bends too. Get the blood moving again. Return to your exam and review it before turning it in.

Have you ever wondered how some students are mysteriously caught cheating? Did you see the hidden camera or microphone? It's there – trust me. If not, just assume it is and behave. Besides if you prepared properly for the exam you will have no need for such behavior, you'll ace the exam.

During high school I struggled – but kept a 3.0 average to get a discount on my auto insurance. Yes, I had to pay for my own insurance. That gave me motivation and an early work ethic. Anyway, when I hit college, I studied my butt off. I had to do this because I wasn't so bright and intelligent as some of the gifted students. I read the material, listened to the class lecture, then reread the material. This three prong approach enabled me to carry a 4.0 throughout college. I told you I'm not so intelligent, but I do know how to work my butt off.

About interviews, get yourself a good book, and practice, practice, practice. You need to be comfortable under fire; the thoughts flow easier. For entry level apprentice type jobs wear a clean shirt and jeans. Anything above that position – Suit and tie. I've sat on interview panels many times. It doesn't impress me when a trainee comes in all decked out. In fact I remember a guy just getting off work. He came in with dirty cloths and a dirty Cowboy hat. He nailed every single question thoroughly, with confidence and energy.

Be sure you don't try to buffalo your way through your

answers. That small exaggeration could cost you. When you say you know how to do something, you better darn well know how to do it. We'll smell it and find out during the interview how much you really know. So instead of saying, I know Electronics or the National Electric Code – it is far better to say, I took a code class a few years ago, I'm probably pretty rusty now, but I did get a " B" in the class. That speaks honesty. Here is another good one: I'm really not good at that procedure, but with proper training, I can work my butt off and learn how to do it properly.

For personal safety equipment type questions – stand up during the interview and start pointing to every part of your body and name the related piece of safety equipment. Go from head to toe.

Sometimes your question has a list be answered, don't stop talking till they tell you to. Answers must be complete and thorough.

Finally, at the end of the interview, shake their hand looking them square in the eyes. A firm solid hand shake, not a bone crusher. You ladies, practice up on that with your father.

The Electricians in the Industry make less than those in the Utilities. You might not be able to quickly get hired into the Utilities, the wait is up to two years sometimes, depending on how high you scored. Take advantage of the IBEW's apprenticeship program. When a Journey

Electrician from the IBEW applies for a High Voltage Position, they command respect and honor.

Why would a Journeyman apply for a training position?

Well the Electrical world has many pieces of pie that make up a whole. Each piece has a specific field of study. They are: Construction, Maintenance, Electronics, Fire Systems, SCADA and High Voltage.

One Journeyman told me, *Why not? You're paying me to go to school!*

Match-Maker

Did you pre-drill those holes before you put those screws in my bones?

"I only used the best carpentry practices," answered my orthopedic surgeon.

Cool, I felt content. Here's a doc who's job was to rebuild my ACL, and he knew, like I did, that if you don't pre-drill the holes, the interference screws will split and splinter the wood.

Family practice physicians are similar to electrical troubleshooters. We both are presented with a machine that is or nearly out of order. We examine the machine, speak with the operator that uses it and find out the abnormal conditions. Now we run our tests. Through a method of logical progression we use our meters to hunt down, locate, and correct our problems. However, being an Electrician is a bit more rewarding, machines don't lie to us, they don't try to sue us, they can always be repaired, and when you walk away from the machine, you know darn good and well that it was fixed 100 percent.

As a child I wanted to be an actor, well teaching is similar to acting. We both research our roles, prepare our scripts and get on stage to deliver the show of a lifetime. We listen to the movie critics, and hopefully do a better job the next time.

Can you see where I'm going with this? Just because your candy is after-dinner mints, doesn't mean that Tic-Tacs aren't just as good.

Oh, I might screw up on some of these. I was taking a night class siting next to an Air-Force fighter pilot. I asked why he was getting his MBA and not flying for the Airlines. He snorted loudly, "WHAT, fly a damn school bus in the air?" I guess he did have his point. Well, please keep an open mind. These are only suggestions not insults. Finally, you don't need to be a physician to show loving kindness, compassion and charity. You can select a job that fits you, then on off hours volunteer in your own city. You don't need to travel abroad to some foreign land. If you open your eyes you will find plenty that needs your help. Volunteering in this manner reaps rewards far greater than volunteering just to get into med school.

Remember all those reasons why you wanted to become a physician? Well, with our infinite wisdom we will attempt to match those reasons to similar jobs in the industry. We will not limit you to High-Voltage work, in-fact some of these may include the medical field – but that all depends on your ego. After we play match maker, we will list those jobs, pay scale, their job hazards, and requirements to apply for the position.

" Master Bruce, why do we fall down?"

So we can learn how to pick ourselves back up!

1.   **Money:** *Electric Service Manager, Port Pilot, System Operator, swing-shift*

2.   **Prestige – Power Status Symbol**:

Having any kind of Doctorate in the upper ranks of management pulls a lot of weight both in and out of the office.

3.   **Surgeon**: Master Chef (Chef de cuisine), Finish Carpenter, Custom made furniture, Saddle Maker

4.   **ER Physician**: System Operator, Firefighter, Transmission Live-line worker

5.   **Dermatology**: Industrial Hygienist, Environmental Health / Safety

6.   **Anesthesiology**: Certified Nurse Anesthetist, Natural gas petrochemical engineer

7.   **Colon and Rectal**: Wastewater treatment Electrician/Plumber

8.   **Gynecology**: Woman's shelter – crisis intervention.

9.   **Pediatrics**: Women's Center Early Childhood teacher

10.   **Plastic Surgery**: Hollywood makeup artists, Movie Latex Monster Mask-Makers

11.   **Radiology**: Electrical utility construction photography and water utility photographers

12.   **Pulmonologist:** Aerospace engineering, NASA, Wind-tunnel Test Engineer

13.   **Teaching**: Industrial Hygienist

14.   **Multi-task-er**: Station Operator, Generating Station Operator

15.   **Mega-Monster Multi-task-er**: System Operator

16.   **The builder:** Construction Electrical Mechanic

17.   **The Cowboy**: Lineman, Electrical Distribution Mechanic, Cable Splicer

18: **Working on steel towers where the birds fly**: Transmission Live Line Worker

19.   **The watch-maker**: Instrument Mechanic

20.   **Testing Mega-Equipment**: Diagnostics, Station Test group (A darn good job, not to dirty, specialists in complex testing to prove electrical equipment, cable and machinery.)

21.   **Excitement:** Transmission Live Line Worker: They climb out of helicopters onto 500,000 volts!

https://www.youtube.com/watch?v=FGoaXZwFlJ4

Wages !

These are the wages of the secret jobs without overtime included. Remember, if it's Utility related – risk goes up, pay goes up.

National Average	West Coast Wages

The **Port Pilot** tops the list of wages $ 400,000 !

$ 227,675

Certified Nurse Anesthetist $ 166,400

$ 190,000

System Operator, *Load Dispatcher,* $ 76,500

$ 145,000

Natural gas petrochemical engineer $ 99,000

$ 145,000

Water Works Engineer $ 54,000

$ 142,000

Engineering Geologist $ 54,000

$ 142,000

Chief Electric Plant Operator $ 86,519

$ 141,000

Systems Programmer $ 86,275	**$ 139,000**
Industrial Hygienist $ 77,770	**$ 122,000**
Lineman Apprentice:	**$60,205 to $94,127**
Lineman Journey-level $ 71,274	**$ 120,707**
Utility Chemist $ 75,530	**$ 119,000**
Water Biologist / Microbiologist $ 54,000	**$ 105,000**
Electrical Mechanic $ 75,500	**$ 102,000**
Station Operator $ 76,580	**$ 102,000**
Chef de cuisine $ 75–100,000	**$ 75 –100,000**

Utility Millwright $ 50,472	$ 100,000
Utility Carpenters $ 67,000	$ 99,000
Utility Plumber $ 50,660	$ 98,000
Utility Painter $ 48,000	$ 95,000
Electrical Tester $ 69,000	$ 91,000
Steam Plant Assistant $ 56,000	$ 80,000
Electrical utility construction photography $ 46,300	$ 78,000

Swing Shift   Usually from 4:00 pm to 12:30 am. An extra 7-10 % more than base wage.

These are the treasure pages of all the top dollar jobs. Remember, top money in a job you can't stand, or that is not a good fit doesn't make sense.

'If it doesn't fit, you must acquit'

Final Thought

I checked online regarding going to school in the Caribbean. I certainly found a couple of hard to get into – demanding Med Schools. I was all ready to write a complete page of how the Caribbean could be a worth while Plan B – but I don't think I can. Recently I went to the Urgent Care, the doc was young, very intelligent, and in my opinion, was pretty darn good. So good, I asked him what Med school he went to. He evasively and quickly answered a nameless school in the Caribbean, this state, that state, finally he said finishing up at UCLA. Having done some research on my own, I tried to pick him up by saying, "Did you go to St. George?" He started to beam, "I went to American University of the Caribbean School of Medicine!"

Well now, his training appeared to be quite competent, however going to school in the Caribbean seemed to be an embarrassment. Kind of like a boy having the name Sue, or Maria. In order to have such names, it forces you to be one tough mean dude, ready to clobber anyone who makes fun of it. Now, if he hung his head with me, odds are that he doesn't socialize much with other physicians...... unless they too graduated from the islands.

However -

Do you have a fondness for India, Yoga, hands on healing, the body mind and Spirit? Go Ayurvedic.

Do you enjoy Tai Chi, Chi Gung, Martial Arts? Go Traditional Chinese Medicine.

The best Ayurveda school in the nation is taught by Dr. Vasant Lad in New Mexico, The Ayurvedic Institute. You have to complete two levels of instruction, to start your practice.... That's two years.

The study of Ayurveda brings you into the information which has been gathered from centuries of day-to-day experiences. From specific points on the body to press and massage, to beneficial herbs and foods that meet the needs of specific body types. You will learn that the same spicy herb is corrective in some body types are not to be given to a Vata body type.

I went to the Institute's website and purchased a few books. If you want just one good book, get this one: Ayurvedic Cooking for Self-Healing by Usha and Vasant Lad, B.A.M.S., M.A.Sc.

There is a Buddhist Monk in Berkeley who chose to study with him for six years. His Buddhist spin on Ayureveda can be found on Archive.org

Be careful in selecting another school. Do your research, find out all the complaints at Yelp and other sites. You might run into Ayurvedic Masters who promise secret methods if you join his tribe. All I can say is it's not a perfect world. There is the good, the bad and the ugly. Before you buy into any Guru, do your research, check his complaint record, dig deep, do a critical evaluation. Things might not be so rosy.

Will you be able to become a Doctor in Ayurvedic medicine? You'll have to complete your studies in India. That Doctorate will not work to well in the US. In fact, it might be pretty darn tough to make a living practicing Ayurveda. So why study it at all? It makes a terrific complement to Traditional Oriental Medicine. The two approaches go hand in hand. I like describing people in the Ayurvedic method: vata , pita, kapha. However I like the Chinese Five element theory over the Ayurvedic element theory. I will say that just by knowing the Ayurevedic approach, I was able to answer some sample State license exam questions for Chinese medicine.

Now, about TCM.

This is a Doctorate Degree in traditional Chinese medicine. Many schools just offer a Master's program. That's because after receiving a MS, you take your board exams and can open up a practice. You can go to the State Licensing board in Acupuncture and download a practice exam.

The site also details what kind of knowledge you will be examined on.

Be sure that the school you select is really accredited, many are not. Look at their stat sheets detailing how many enrolled each year, and how many graduated. There was a few very impressive web sites – yet they had horrible stats. Some are not colleges as advertised, just clinics. I found Emperor's College very impressive.

"Emperor's is widely recognized as having the finest faculty in the U.S. and among the top 5 in the world."

Be sure to completely review Emperor's course catalog. Don't be afraid to click way up on top of the main web page in the covert black area. Find Current Students – now explore! (check out the syllabus section)

After a MS in TCM you will have a complete understanding of every acupuncture point on the body, know about 250 Chinese herbs, tongue colors, pulse diagnosis, and how the inner spirit works.

You will learn Chinese characters, but just the medical ones, not the super hard stuff.

What's really great about this course of study is that you can specialize in Pediatrics, Gynecology or Dermatology. You know all that anatomy and physiology you already studied? You'll breeze through the first year of studies here. After you get the MS, Stay for another two years to get the Doctorate.

The DAOM program at Emperor's College consists of

1,250 total hours – 600 hours of didactic instruction and 650 hours of advanced clinical rotations – completed over the course of eight academic quarters.

They offer a dual-specialization in Internal Medicine & Physical Medicine.

Doctoral fellows receive clinical and didactic training in all areas of the Internal Medicine specialty:

- Cardiology
- Reproductive Medicine
- Oncology
- Immunology I

Physical Medicine Specialty

- Orthopedics
- Sports Medicine
- Stroke Rehabilitation & Prevention

Job prospects are greater in this field than Ayurvedic Medicine. Many HMO's have TCM Doctors on staff. Both Ayurvedic and TCM schools teach preventive medicine, healing the mind, body and spirit.

This is not just rubbing marma points or sticking needles in people.

Some philosophies view a Doctor as a Priest, and a Priest as a Doctor. If this sounds like you, then this is a terrific start to that path.

Conclusion

Working for the utilities make a terrific Plan B.

I did say work.

Most jobs that work on or near energized equipment are highly dangerous.

But with proper training, guarding against complacency, you can have a wonderful life near the one percent-ers.

Please go back now and read the Preface before continuing.

Thank You,

I wish you immeasurable blessings in you search.

Peter A. J.

Appendix A

Apprenticeship Programs

(excerpts from their web page)

Union Apprenticeship Programs are an excellent place to get jump-start a career. Remember that Silver Tsunami I told you about? Well, I'm pretty sure it applies to all the trades. So, here is a job that pays you to work in the field and attend their trade specific school. A word of caution: Non-union school credits are not accepted at union schools. So, think good and hard if you want to pay good money to attend one of those. Work Union – get paid better, and work safer.

IBEW: The IBEW represents approximately 750,000 active members and retirees who work in a wide variety of fields, including utilities, construction, telecommunications, broadcasting, manufacturing, railroads and government.

LOCAL 532 Texas

OUTSIDE LINE APPRENTICESHIP PROGRAM
Inside Apprenticeship

http://ibew532.com/currentaffair/?page_id=24

UA: The United Association of Journeymen and Apprentices of the Plumbing and Pipe Fitting Industry of the United States, Canada (UA), affiliated with the national building trades, represents approximately 340,000 plumbers, pipefitters, sprinkler fitters, service technicians and welders in local unions across North America. The UA has been training qualified pipe tradesmen and women longer than anyone else in the industry.

Millwright: The person who works with his hands is a laborer; the person that works with his hands and his head is an artisan; the person who works with his hands, his head and his heart is a Union Millwright. A millwright is a trades person who installs, maintains and repairs stationary industrial machinery and mechanical equipment by interpreting drawings, performing layouts and assembling parts until they are in perfect working order. Construction millwrights and industrial mechanics work in a variety of industries, and can pursue complementary training and develop additional skills in steel fabrication, welding, machining, electronics, hydraulics or pneumatics.

Boilermaker: The International Brotherhood of Boilermakers is a diverse union representing workers throughout the United States and Canada in industrial construction, repair, and maintenance; manufacturing; shipbuilding and marine repair; railroads; mining and quarrying; cement kilns; and related industries

Carpenters: The CITF and its affiliated training programs invest more than $200 million a year to develop and deliver training for U3C members. Through a network of more than 200 training centers across North America and 2,500 full-time instructors, UBC members can learn today's in-demand skills at little or no out-of-pocket expense.

Lineman: *http://www.calnevjatc.org* Apprentice linemen assist the journeymen linemen in building and maintaining electrical power systems. The apprenticeship program at California-Nevada JATC combines supervised, structured on-the-job training with related classroom instruction to prepare you for skilled employment within the industry. Because you are working and learning at the same time, apprentices are considered full-time employees. Wages are paid to you during the on-the-job phase of training. Wages increase as progress is made in the program.

Apprentice Communications Tech. PG& E: The Apprentice Communication Technician is responsible for assisting qualified Journeyman Technicians in installing, testing, retiring or removing the following equipment: microwave radios with antennas and transmission lines; data, telemetry and supervisory systems, construct, enhance and maintain computer and telephone network systems by assembling parts and equipment and executing the job design package.

Cal Dept of Water Resources:
http://www.water.ca.gov/apprenticetraining/

The Department of Water Resources Operations and Maintenance Training Center is the gateway to a career as a: Hydroelectric Plant Electrician, Hydroelectric Plant Mechanic, Hydroelectric Plant Operator, Utility Crafts Worker

Port Pilot: US Merchant Marines:
http://www.usmma.edu/

Academy graduates abide by the motto "Acta Non Verba" - deeds not words, and are leaders that exemplify the concept of service above self. Employers like to hire Kings Point graduates because of their leadership abilities, self-discipline, practical experience, problem-solving skills and professional expertise. Virtually 100 percent of our graduates obtain well-paying employment within six months of commencement – with the majority at work within three months, and most with offers of employment before graduation day. The piloting profession is widely considered the pinnacle of a maritime career. The first step to becoming a pilot is to first be a professional mariner with drive and determination. There is no direct path. There are no "pilot" schools or any training system that takes a totally unfamiliar person off the street and turns them into a maritime pilot. Some pilots have had careers on ocean-going vessels and others had careers on inland vessels such as tugs and barges.

City of San Francisco – Water, Power, Sewer:

This place has a boatload of apprenticeship programs
http://www.sfwater.org/index.aspx?page=888

Appendix B

Schools:

In case some of these schools are impacted. Do not let that stop you from finding another in a different city or state. You may have to live with an Aunt or Uncle out of town for awhile.

(excerpts from their course catalog)

Lansing Community College (LCC) : Michigan
http://www.lcc.edu/utility/lineworker/

Electrical Utility Lineworker Program

Once you have been accepted into the program, you will complete 13 months of intensive coursework consisting of a four day Utility Lineworker orientation, three semesters of academic courses, and a 9-Week climbing school conducted at a utility training center. Successful completion of this program will prepare you to enter lineworker apprenticeships with utility companies, or other occupations that require similar skills.

Northwest Lineman College
https://www.lineman.edu/programs/

Since 1993, Northwest Lineman College has provided various elements of power delivery training to over 2000 individuals from across the US and Canada. We continually strive to have our programs achieve the benchmark standard of training. Our mission of delivering this benchmark standard of training is centered on three key objectives:

•Delivering training that will provide the foundation for starting a long and exciting career in the power delivery industry for individuals new to the industry.
•Delivering training that will result in employees in the power delivery industry becoming more knowledgeable, skillful, and valuable to their employers.
•Contributing to the evolution of the industry by developing and providing various products that enhance safety and productivity.

Currently, the most popular training programs we offer are our Electrical Lineworker Program (ELP) and our Lineworker Certification Program (LCP previously known as the Power Delivery Program):

➜   Electrical Lineworker Program
➜   Utility Training Services
➜   Lineworker Certification Program

Powerline Mechanic Training Program: Los Angeles Trade Tech
http://college.lattc.edu/cmu/program/electrical-lineman-training-program/

Development of basic skills needed to be successful trainees for electrical-related career ladders are emphasized. These skills include: overall safety considerations, power pole climbing skills, knowledge of the basic tools and materials involved with the electrical line crafts, general construction standards, basic rigging principles, and basic electrical theory that is specific to this trade. A 175 hour power pole-climbing certificate of completion is granted to students who successfully complete the course. A component of this course also includes preparation for Civil Service examinations that are likely required for positions at municipal companies.

Los Angeles Trade-Technical College offers various programs for individuals interested in working in the utility industry. The programs enable individuals to be prepared to take the entry level certification for electrical craft helper and entry in to various Utility Lineman Apprentice Program such as: DWP, SCE, SG&E, PG&E. It is recommended to begin with the fundamentals certificate of achievement and then move to the larger certificates and then complete the degree programs. The certificates are stack-able meaning as you reach each level the classes build so you do not have to repeat courses that you have already taken.

Tennessee Valley Public power Association
http://www.tvppa.com/Pages/training/certificate.aspx

Click on Lineman Apprentice

Stark State College / Ohio Edison   Line Worker Technician Major *http://www.starkstate.edu/academic-programs/line-worker-tech*

Stark State College Substation Worker Technician Major *http://www.starkstate.edu/academic-programs/substation-worker-tech*

Ohio Edison, a subsidiary of FirstEnergy Corp. (NYSE: FE), is partnering with Stark State College to reinstate its award-winning program to train the next generation of utility line and substation workers.

The Power Systems Institute is a two-year program that combines learning hands-on utility skills at an Ohio Edison training facility with technical coursework learned in a Stark State College classroom. Program graduates will earn an Associate of Applied Science degree with a focus on electric power utility technology.

"The Power Systems Institute already has provided Ohio Edison with nearly 320 highly qualified employees who are working in the field today, using the training they received from this unique program to help keep the lights on for our customers," said Randall A. Frame, regional president of Ohio Edison. "Whether it's linemen who work above ground or substation personnel who operate on the ground, PSI provides great training for someone looking for a career in the utility industry."

MEDICAL / HEALTH RELATED SCHOOLING

Industrial Hygienist: Environmental and Occupational Health Cal State University Northridge

With well over 200 majors, we are the largest accredited EOH program in the nation. These numbers are essential for addressing the unfolding workforce crisis in environmental and occupational health. In terms of total numbers, we are also the most diverse accredited EOH program in the nation. In a profession that values our ability to communicate with the public, diversity matters. Our mission is to develop the very best EOH practitioners in the field. We pursue various lines of research, teaching, and service towards that end. Our graduates have earned doctoral and professional degrees all over the nation and, more importantly, attained leadership levels in virtually every area of our profession. We are fortunate to be located in a major academic center for EOH, and we value our many connections with other universities and related agencies. Six full-time faculty members, along with numerous affiliated and part-time faculty, presently teach in the Department of Environmental and Occupational Health (EOH). The program emphasizes the study of the chemical, physical and biological factors that affect human health and environmental quality. The curriculum provides the basic knowledge and training required for professional careers in the field of community environmental health and industrial hygiene.

Certified Nurse Anesthetist:

University of Pittsburgh

Pitt Nursing's Nurse Anesthesia major is ranked FIRST! (2016 US News)

Nurse Anesthesia is one of the Master's options in the School of Nursing. Nurse Anesthesia practice is based on a continuum of care beginning with preoperative assessment and culminating with discharge from the recovery area. Nurse anesthetists interview and assess each patient and formulate and implement a plan of care to best meet individual needs. Throughout the preoperative period, nurse anesthetists serve as patient advocates, provide emotional support, and collaborate with other health care practitioners to provide the optimum anesthetic experience. The University of

Pittsburgh School of Nursing's, Nurse Anesthesia curriculum prepares registered nurses for entry into anesthesia practice. Graduates are prepared to administer a full range of anesthetics to a wide variety of patients across the lifespan. Through an integrated process of classroom and clinical instruction, students develop the didactic knowledge base and clinical skills necessary for safe and effective practice. Students rotate through numerous clinical sites in Pittsburgh, the surrounding region, and now more distant sites to enhance clinical experiences. The University of Pittsburgh Medical Center (UPMC) Health System hospitals are world renowned in the areas of surgical innovation, trauma medicine, organ transplantation, research, and biomedical technology. Rotations including specialized experiences in cardiothoracic, neurosurgical, dental, regional anesthesia, organ transplantation, pediatrics, obstetrics, burns and electroconvulsive therapy enrich the curriculum. Clinical rotations in community hospitals help to broadly prepare the graduate for practice in diverse settings. Students work directly with nationally and internationally renowned leaders in research, practice, and education. Upon completion, graduates are well prepared to safely manage simple to extremely complex patients. Nurse Anesthesia coursework is offered in a full time format over 28 months and classes begin each August and January. Part-time study is also available for the core curriculum. Clinical practice begins as two days/week in the first term and increases in both intensity and frequency throughout the course of study. Clinical in is the final two terms is 4-5 days/week and is interspersed with clinical conferences and preparation sessions for the Certification Examination. Nurse Anesthesia considers registered nurses with a minimum of 1 year of full-time critical care nursing experience and a BSN degree. Academic transcripts, professional references, GRE examination results, and an essay must be submitted to be considered for an interview with faculty. The Nurse Anesthesia MSN and Post-Masters DNP programs are accredited through 2019 by the American Association of Nurse Anesthetists Council on Accreditation of Nurse Anesthesia Educational Programs. Graduates of the MSN Program are eligible to take the National Certification Examination administered by the National Board for Certification and Recertification of Nurse Anesthetists (NBCRNA). Students are accepted from a wide variety of critical care backgrounds and with a variety of career goals. Registered nurses who do not have a BSN may enroll via the RN Options choosing the RN-MSN path.

Certified Nurse Anesthetist:

Baylor College of Medicine Graduate Program in Nurse Anesthesia The Baylor College of Medicine Graduate Program in Nurse Anesthesia is committed to the promotion of excellence in the nurse anesthesia profession through education, research, and healthcare. The Graduate Program in Nurse Anesthesia provides a comprehensive graduate learning experience for registered nurses in the practice of administering all forms of anesthesia in preparation for assuming roles as qualified nurse anesthetists. The 36-month program culminates in a Doctor of Nursing Practice degree from Baylor College of Medicine. The program is divided into two phases: an 18-month didactic experience and an 18-month clinical practicum. The didactic phase consists of coursework in the basic and clinical sciences, healthcare delivery and policy, translational research, leadership and management. The clinical phase provides extensive clinical education in the provision of general, regional, and local anesthesia. Upon completion of the degree requirements, graduates are eligible to take the National Certification Examination administered by the National Board on Certification and Recertification of Nurse Anesthetists. The College also offers advanced standing in the DNP program for master's-prepared Certified Registered Nurse Anesthetists who wish to pursue a doctoral degree. CRNAs with advanced standing complete the required coursework in 24 months. The schedule of classes is designed to accommodate working professionals. Most courses are offered in an online format with limited on-campus time required. Upon completion of the program, CRNAs will receive a DNP degree.

Certified Nurse Anesthetist:

USC Program of Nurse Anesthesia/Keck School of Medicine The USC Program of Nurse Anesthesia offers an intense academic and comprehensive clinical curriculum. Students will gain experience in a variety of clinical specialty areas including general, cardiothoracic, neurosurgical, genitourinary, gynecologic, head and neck, plastic, orthopedic, trauma, burns, transplantation, robotics, obstetric, pediatric and outpatient procedures. Students have the most sophisticated anesthesia equipment at their disposal. Under the guidance of expert CRNA and physician faculty primarily provided by the Keck School of Medicine/Department of Anesthesiology faculty, student nurse anesthetists are responsible for the administration and management of general anesthesia, regional anesthetic techniques and modalities of invasive monitoring. Students also receive experience in acute and chronic pain management. The Program offers an optional Specialty Fellowship in a variety of anesthesia specialties. Clinical instruction is offered in numerous state of the art medical centers in Southern California. The ratio of students to faculty is usually 1:1 and never exceeds 2:1.

Clinical instruction is provided by both CRNAs and physician anesthesiologists. By graduation, students must have provided anesthesia services for at least 550 cases and are expected to manage all aspects of perioperative care. The graduate students' academic and clinical curriculum includes simulation in the USC Program of Nurse Anesthesia Simulation Center. High-fidelity simulation encompasses basic and advanced principles and performance assessment is formatted to the students' level of training. Students will be prepared to become a valued member of the anesthesia care team and develop critical thinking skills that far exceed minimum standards for entry level practice. Graduates of the Program are academically and clinically prepared to provide quality anesthesia care to meet the health care needs of the community and its diverse population. Upon completion of all clinical and academic requirements, graduates are eligible to take the national certification examination given by the National Board on Certification and Re-certification of Nurse Anesthetists.

Appendix C

Requirements and Job Descriptions.

https://www.governmentjobs.com/careers/lacity/classspecs

There's plenty at this web site, but here are the ones I picked out for you.

APPRENTICE MACHINIST

One year of full-time paid experience as a mechanical helper in the mechanical or metal trades; <u>and</u>

Six months of coursework in machine tool training at a high school or trade school level. Six months of coursework is equivalent to one semester or two quarter courses.

An Apprentice Machinist works as an apprentice under close supervision, assisting journey-level machinists and receiving on-the-job instruction in using precision hand and machine tools in the repair, rebuilding, and dismantling, fabrication, and installation of machinery and equipment.

APPRENTICE METAL TRADES

One year of full-time paid experience as a helper in the mechanical or metal trades; <u>and</u>

Six months of coursework in a metal trade at the high school or trade school level.

Six months of coursework is equivalent to one semester or two quarter courses.

An Apprentice-Metal Trades works as an apprentice in a specific metal trade, receives on-the-job training assisting a journey-level Sheet Metal Worker, Structural Steel Shop Worker, Blacksmith, Welder, or Auto Body Builder and Repairer; attends approved classroom instruction during off duty hours.

ASSISTANT ELECTRICAL TESTER

Completion of one course in Chemistry, Physics, or Electricity from a high school or trade school.

An Assistant Electrical Tester makes routine calibration tests of watt-hour meters, makes routine electrical tests of materials and electrical appliances and assists in testing more complex electric instruments and equipment.

BOAT CAPTAIN

Current employment with the City of Los Angeles; and Three years of full-time paid experience in the operation of inboard motor boats on large bodies of water.

A Boat Captain operates a single engine and/or twin

engine diesel-powered seagoing boat transporting port pilots at the Port of Los Angeles and personnel doing marine and environmental monitoring and research, towing pile-driving and work barges to various work locations, or operating a tour boat at the Port of Los Angeles; may perform minor maintenance on marine diesel engines; may supervise staff involved in the above activities; applies sound supervisory principles and techniques in building and maintaining an effective work force; and does related work.

CARPENTER

Completion of a recognized apprenticeship as a carpenter or cabinetmaker; or

Six years of full-time paid experience performing carpenter or cabinetmaker work.

A Carpenter does skilled rough and finish carpentry in building and repairing wood structures and articles.

CHEMIST

Graduation from a recognized four-year college or university with a major in Chemistry, Chemical Engineering or Biochemistry, with course work or experience utilizing at least two of the following instruments:

1. Gas Chromatograph

2. Atomic Absorption Spectrophotometer

3. Fourier Transform Infrared Spectrometer

4. Ion Chromatograph

5. High-performance Liquid Chromatograph

6. Inductively Coupled Plasma Spectrometer

7. Mass Spectrometer

8. Hand-held or automated: laboratory or field sampling and monitoring equipment

9 Multi-element Oil Analyzer

10. X-Ray Fluorescence Spectrometer

A Chemist performs difficult organic, inorganic and physical chemical analyses and research studies in connection with water quality, wastewater, storm water, solid resources and industrial water treatment, construction and maintenance materials, arson investigations, expert testimony, and hazardous waste assessments; conducts tests and experimental work in relation to the measurement of air and water quality and the control of combustion products; researches, evaluates, and summarizes scientific literature; prepares standard operating procedures for using laboratory and field instruments; reviews test results and prepares technical reports; follows quality assurance and safety programs and performs routine maintenance of analytical instruments; may collect water and sediment samples in the field; may review and analyze scientific reports and data related to environmental assessment, water quality, and public health; and may prepare written conclusions and recommendations.

CIVIL ENGINEERING ASSOCIATE

Graduation from a recognized four-year college or university with a degree in engineering, which includes at least 24 semester units or 36 quarter units of core courses in civil engineering; <u>or</u>

Possession of a valid Engineer-In-Training Certificate recognized by the State of California Board for Professional Engineers and Land Surveyors.

A Civil Engineering Associate performs professional civil engineering work in researching, checking, computing, conducting field work needed, and working with consultants in the preparation of plans, designs, details, specifications, cost estimates, environmental documentation, and various reports for the construction, maintenance, and operation of a wide variety of civil engineering projects; processes private development plans and development actions; issues engineering permits to the public; and does related work.

ELECTRIC DISTRIBUTION MECHANIC TRAINEE

ELECTRIC DISTRIBUTION MECHANIC (Lineman)

This is the Cowboy Job, which you can then promote into Line Patrol Mechanic

ELECTRIC STATION OPERATOR

An Electric Station Operator must successfully complete a two-year intensive on-the-job and classroom training program in order to receive an appointment to a regular Electric Station Operator position.

An Electric Station Operator operates high voltage electric and auxiliary equipment in hydroelectric generating, receiving and distributing stations and in high voltage DC Converter Plants; performs routine inspections, meter readings, and cleaning of high voltage equipment and facilities; and does other related duties.

ELECTRICAL ENGINEERING ASSISTANT

Current employment with the City of Los Angeles in a regular part-time or full-time position; and

2.   Graduation from a school of Engineering in a recognized four-year college or university with a degree in Engineering, which includes at least 24 semester units or 36 quarter units of Electrical Engineering core courses. Course work in the following is highly desirable, but not required: circuit analysis, electronics, electric machines, power transmission, and control systems; or

3.   Possession of a valid Engineer-in-Training Certificate recognized by the California State Board of Registration for Professional Engineers; or

4.   College seniors who expect to graduate by September. 1993, from a school of

Engineering in a recognized four-year college or university may apply. However, you cannot be appointed until you have completed all your course work, and the, 24 semester units or 36 quarter units described in Requirement NO.2.

5.   All candidates must attach to the application a supplemental form containing a list of the Electrical Engineering core courses completed, detailing the name of the school, course, credit earned, and grade received.

An Electrical Engineering Assistant does professional work in preparing electrical engineering designs, reports, plans, specifications, calculations, estimates and computer programs; and testing and inspection activities related to the manufacturing, construction, installation, operation, and maintenance of power and/or other 'electrical and electronic equipment and systems.

ELECTRICAL ENGINEERING DRAFTING TECHNICIAN

Completion of 12 semester units or 18 quarter units in drafting, including at least 6 semester units or 9 quarter units in electrical drafting; and 6 semester units or 9 quarter units in mathematics at a recognized college, trade or technical school; or

Two years of full-time paid engineering drafting experience, one year of which was in electrical engineering drafting.

An Electrical Engineering Drafting Technician performs responsible subprofessional engineering work and drafting in the preparation of electrical and communication design drawings, wiring diagrams, plans, and charts relating to the construction, operation, and maintenance of a wide variety of electrical installations and facilities.

ELECTRICAL TESTER

Six months of full-time paid experience and current employment as a helper or trainee for a utility performing work on equipment and circuits, construction and maintenance; or

2.   Completion of eight months in the Utility Pre-Craft Trainee training program sponsored by the Los Angeles Department of Water and Power; or

3.   Successful completion of three semester units or four quarter units from a recognized college or university or trade school in physics, chemistry, electricity, or electronics; or

4.   Successful completion of the Pre-Electrical Craft Helper training course presented by the Los

Angeles Trade Technical College.

An entry-level Electrical Tester receives intensive classroom and on-the-job instruction and training. The trainee is supervised by a Senior Electrical Tester and works as a trainee assisting journey-level electrical workers within the Testing Laboratories in the performance of diagnostic tests, calibration, repair, maintenance, and adjustments on: high and low voltage electrical circuits, equipment and related material; meters, smart-grid systems, conventional and renewable generation resources, control circuits, instruments, relays and related equipment and materials; new locations; and performs related duties. A journey-level Electrical Tester: performs routine calibration tests of meters; makes routine electrical tests of material; assists in testing more complex electric instruments and equipment; tests and replaces electric meters, control and protective relays, instruments, transformers, and other equipment and materials; performs cathodic protection in underground and above head structures; performs infrared inspection of high voltage overhead distribution systems; and builds and test circuit boards, removes or replaces components, and tests communication levels, in regard to facility/substation Supervisory Control and Data Acquisition (SCADA) systems, Remote Terminal Units (RTU), and other control systems. Journey-level Electrical Testers may also: lead a group of employees engaged in field or laboratory electrical testing; perform the more difficult and advanced functions of electrical testing; and perform related duties.

ENVIRONMENTAL ASSOCIATE

Graduation from a recognized four-year college or university with a degree in environmental, ecological, biological, chemical, atmospheric or earth science, oceanography, environmental policy, urban planning or a related field, with at least 12 semester -units or 18 quarter units in environmental studies, such as ecology, water pollution, environmental laws and environmental impact analysis. Specific courses, units, and school must be listed in the appropriate box on the application.

An Environmental Associate reviews and analyzes proposed legislation, policies, programs, construction and other projects, and a wide variety of other matters to determine ,their environmental impact on the city; makes recommendations in accordance with established environmental policy and relevant technical information; implements environmental compliance programs; conducts site inspections as necessary; prepares environmental permits; ard assists in the technical management of grant projects and other environmental programs.

ENVIRONMENTAL ENGINEERING ASSOCIATE

Graduation from a recognized four-year college or university with a degree in engineering, which includes at least 12 semester units or 18 quarter units of core courses in sanitary engineering; or

2.   Possession of a valid Engineer-In-Training Certificate recognized by the California State Board of Registration for Professional Engineers.

An Environmental Engineering Associate performs professional sanitary and environmental engineering work in connection with water supp_y, water quality control, solid waste and wastewater collection, disposal and treatment, and ionizing radiation; conducts engineering, planning and research studies in connection with water and solid resources related activities; coordinates construction and operations of water and wastewater treatment and solid waste facilities; and does related work.

INDUSTRIAL HYGIENIST

Graduation from a recognized four-year college or university with a bachelor's degree in Industrial Hygiene, Environmental and Occupational Health, or Safety Engineering; <u>OR</u>

2.   Graduation from a recognized four-year college or university with a bachelor's degree in a related field, such as Biological Science, Physics, or Chemistry, and two years of full-time paid professional experience in an Industrial Hygiene or Safety position involving investigation of environmental hazards, such as air contamination, noise and radiation, and their effect on employees.

An Industrial Hygienist plans, develops, and implements an Industrial Hygiene and Health and Safety Training Program to minimize risk of employee exposure to hazardous chemical and physical stressors in the work environment; identifies significant workplace health hazards, evaluates the risk of injury or illness, and recommends corrective actions; develops policies consistent with State and Federal occupational health and safety laws and advises management regarding solutions to health and safety in the work environment; and assists in implementation of those solutions.

LOAD DISPATCHER / SYSTEM OPERATOR

Two years of full-time paid experience as an electric station operator, steam plant operator, electric distribution mechanic, electrical mechanic, hydroelectric station operator, senior electrical repairer, lineman, senior electrical tester, electric trouble dispatcher or in a position which is at least at that level and provides experience in operating a switchboard controlling the function or maintenance of electric equipment and lines in an electric power generating plant, substation, or in a receiving, switching, or distribution station; or maintaining an electrical distribution system at 4-kV or higher; or

2.   Two years of full-time paid experience as a load dispatcher, systems operator, or in a position which is at least at that level and provides experience in centralized control over electric transmission lines, distribution lines, generating equipment, and/or other electrical equipment of an electric utility system at 4-kV or higher; or

3.   Three years of full-time paid experience in a position at least at the level of electrical engineering associate, which provides experience in power system field operations in maintenance of power system

control equipment, or the functioning or maintenance of electric equipment and lines in an electric power generating plant, in a substation, receiving, switching or distribution station, or maintaining an electrical distribution system at 4-kV or higher voltage and possessing either an Engineer-in-Training certification or a Professional Engineers license; or

4.   Five years of full-time paid experience, including time spent in training, in the operation or maintenance of a nuclear power plant and/or its associated auxiliaries on a naval ship.

There are three phases of training. A one-time bonus of up to $7,500 will be paid to trainees in 3 payments as each phase is completed.

2.   Employees regularly assigned to positions for shifts beginning at or after 2:00 p.m. but before 9:00 p.m. are paid up to an additional 4 percent for each hour worked during any such normal shift.

3.   Employees regularly assigned to positions for shifts beginning at or after 9:00 p.m. but before 4:00 a.m. are paid up to an additional 7 percent for each hour worked during any such normal shift.

A Load Dispatcher exercises, or participates in, centralized control over electric transmission and distribution lines and generating and other electrical equipment of an electrical system, directs switching to remove lines and equipment from service for routine or emergency work, coordinates restoration of service, coordinates and executes the purchase, sale and scheduling of electrical energy and associated services in accordance with contracts and prearranged and real-time schedules, and other related duties.

PORT PILOT

Three years of full-time paid experience as a United States Coast Guard licensed Master or Chief Mate of an inspected vessel, of not less than 5,000 gross tons, on the waters of any ocean; or

2.   Three years of full-time paid experience as a port pilot whose duties include docking and undocking of oceangoing or coastwise vessels in a major port of the United States; or

3.   Three years of full-time paid experience as a Master of a tugboat within the confines of San Pedro Bay and its tributaries, including experience as a Docking Master on flat tow vessels of at least 5,000 gross tons.

All entry level Paygrade I positions are temporary training positions. Employment in such positions is limited to two years during which time incumbents must qualify for advancement to the Port Pilot II level.

SENIOR CHEMIST

Two years of full-time paid professional experience as a Chemist or in a class at least at that level performing a variety of chemical tests in a laboratory.

A Master's degree from a recognized college or university in Chemistry, Environmental Engineering, Environmental Science, Biochemistry, Organic Chemistry or a closely related field, may be substituted for one year of the required experience.

A Senior Chemist supervises the work of a group of Chemists and Laboratory Technicians and participates in performing difficult organic, inorganic, and physical chemical analysis and research studies in connection with water quality, wastewater, air emissions, solid waste, and industrial waste treatment; determines and establishes methods and procedures to be followed in conducting research programs; may assist in directing the activities of a small chemistry laboratory; applies sound supervisory principles and techniques in building and maintaining an effective work force; fulfills equal employment opportunity responsibilities; and does related work.

WATER BIOLOGIST

Graduation from a recognized four-year college or university with completion of 24 semester or 36 quarter units in biology, marine biology, botany or zoology. Courses in algology, bacteriology, chemistry, ecology, environmental sciences, invertebrate zoology, limnology, microbiology, oceanography and statistics are desirable.

In addition to the regular application form, each candidate is required to complete an application supplement entitled Water Biologist Application Supplement that details the candidate's technical background and experience.

A Water Biologist performs oceanographic, marine biological, estuarine, limnological, stormwater, freshwater, and wetland surveys; conducts analyses of marine, estuarine, and freshwater aquatic organisms; performs toxicological tests using marine and freshwater organisms; performs biological activated sludge analysis on wastewater; assesses the impact of wastewater and stormwater discharges; identifies marine and freshwater invertebrates, fish, algae and vegetation; collects physical, chemical and biological data in water reservoirs and tanks for maintaining water quality; researches and develops new water quality equipment and processes; conducts studies;

analyzes and writes reports on biological and associated data; reviews and comments on pertinent documents; confers with governmental agencies on water quality matters; represent the City at meetings and conferences; and may act as lead worker or supervisor for employees engaged in performing such tasks.

WATER MICROBIOLOGIST

Graduation from a recognized four-year college or university with a degree in Microbiology or Bacteriology;<u>or</u>

Graduation from a recognized four-year university or college with 24 semester or 36 quarter units in any combination of Microbiology, Bacteriology, Parasitology, Virology, Microbial Ecology, Microbial Physiology, Mycology, Biochemistry, Public Health, or Statistics.

In addition to the regular City application, each candidate must complete and submit the Water Microbiologist Application Supplement at the time of filing. Candidates who fail to submit these documents within the time required will not be considered further in this examination and their applications will not be processed.

A Water Microbiologist uses a variety of

microbiological methods and techniques in performing special studies of microbiological activities which affect the City's water system; prepares reports and recommendations on the impact of such activity on water quality and/or public safety; researches and develops improvements in analyzing bacteria, protozoa, viruses and other microorganisms; and may direct technical employees engaged in routine microbiological tests.

Appendix D

In this appendix you will find the career opportunities page for the various utilities near you.

Start here first: *http://www.energycentraljobs.com/*

Alabama:

http://www.alabamapower.com/about-us/career.asp

California:

http://www.edison.com/home/careers.html

http://cityofpasadena.net/waterandpower/jobs/

https://www.burbankwaterandpower.com/employment jobs-at-bwp

https://www.governmentjobs.com/careers/lacity

http://careers.pge.com/

https://www.smud.org/en/about-smud/careers/working-at-smud/jobs/

Florida:

http://www.nexteraenergy.com/careers/

Georgia:

http://www.georgiapower.com/in-your-community/cool-jobs/home.cshtml

http://www.southerncompany.com/about-us/careers/home.cshtml

Illinois:

http://www.exeloncorp.com/peopleandculture/opportunities/overview.aspx

New Jersey:

https://sjobs.brassring.com/en/asp/tg/cim_advsearch.asp?partnerid=467&siteid=212

New York:

CON EDISON VERY IMPRESSIVE !!!!
http://apps.coned.com/careers/careers/jobs.asp

On this Web page you will find a list of the largest electrical Utility in your own state

https://en.wikipedia.org/wiki/List_of_United_States_electric_companies

List of United States water companies

https://en.wikipedia.org/wiki/List_of_United_States_water_companies

Youtube videos to give you insight for the job of:

Lineman:
https://www.youtube.com/watch?v=FhrRS4LPhNI
https://www.youtube.com/watch?v=B-K5bDs7GFA
https://www.youtube.com/watch?v=WKm3s0NwTrI

Substation Electrician:
https://www.youtube.com/watch?v=BWzhM9tphRk
https://www.youtube.com/watch?v=KgOYNrqoJ58

Station Test Group:
https://www.youtube.com/watch?v=RTeTKpTa0cA
https://www.youtube.com/watch?v=4L0ch0-Paq8

The links are case sensitive.